PREGNANCY & PARENTING

A COMPLETE GUIDE FOR FIRST TIME PARENTS ON PREGNANCY, CHILDBIRTH AND NEWBORN CARE

2-BOOK BUNDLE

BY HELEN WHITE

Respective authors own all copyrights not held by the publisher.

The information herein is offered for informational purposes solely, and is universal as so. The presentation of the information is without contract or any type of guarantee assurance.

The trademarks that are used are without any consent, and the publication of the trademark is without permission or backing by the trademark owner. All trademarks and brands within this book are for clarifying purposes only and are the owned by the owners themselves, not affiliated with this document.

Disclaimer

PARENTING

EVERYTHING YOU NEED TO KNOW BEFORE HAVING A BABY

BY HELEN WHITE

TABLE OF CONTENTS

Table of Contents...6

Introduction..7

Chapter 1: Marriage and Relationships.................................9

Chapter 2: Communication 18

Chapter 3: Other Relationships in Your Life 21

Chapter 4: Finances...26

Chapter 5: Emotions..33

Chapter 6: Timing..39

Chapter 7: Pregnancy 43

Chapter 8: The Caregiver Rule 47

Chapter 9: Discipline—the Rules 50

Chapter 10: Housing and Stability 53

Chapter 11: Work and Stability 56

Conclusion 59

INTRODUCTION

Children make you smile, laugh, cry, and experience numerous other emotions from the minute they are born till the end of your life. It is an amazing experience to raise a child or more than one child, knowing you have done your best to raise an adult you can love, and be proud of.

When you accept the responsibility of raising a child, you are accepting that you are going to put their needs first for the next 18 years, at least. Your life is no longer your own to do what you wish all the time.

It will take an adjustment, and preparedness to get you ready to truly accept your new responsibilities. It is best if you can prepare for your decision to have children, but you may not be able to. You may already be pregnant and full of excitement about your soon to be motherhood. You may be the expectant father, too, and hope to find some information about parenting that can help you prepare in the months you have left before your adorable child's arrival.

The intention of the information included in these chapters is to help you prepare for children, mostly while you are still in the thought and planning stage. However, there will be some information for parents who are already expecting their first child.

There are aspects of your life that you will need to get ready. Parents who take the time to think, plan and prepare are better prepared for the rocky, but loving road ahead of them. Plenty of worries are probably already swirling around in your mind.

What if I say the wrong thing? What if I don't recognize an illness in my child? What happens if my child is born with a disability or illness? What if my child is smarter than me and I can't help them with their homework? You can ask all the what ifs in the world, but sometimes there are things you will not be able to prepare for.

There are two things you need to always keep in mind when it comes to raising a happy baby who becomes a happy child: love and affectionate displays.

You need to show your child you love them, not just say the words. You need to provide hugs and kisses to your child daily, whether or not they have done something you are proud of. Your child should never grow up doubting your love and affection. They should not be afraid to receive and give hugs, or afraid to say "I love you."

If you can provide your baby and growing child with love and affectionate displays, they will grow up happy. They will grow up seeing the value of the lessons you have taught them.

CHAPTER 1:

MARRIAGE AND RELATIONSHIPS

Raising a well-adjusted, happy, and loved baby is in part about the stability you can provide your child. There is a general perception of what is normal and best for children. In recent years, this norm is being challenged. It is not about how you form a marriage or relationship with your partner that matters. You may not have a partner, but have plenty of love to give a child you bear and raise. The key is the stability you provide and making certain your child doesn't feel as though there is anything missing in their life.

An aunt has told her nieces this from time to time, "it hurts that life is not the same. It is confusing and painful that your parents are divorced. But, you need to look on the bright side. You still have two parents in your life. There are children who don't have a mother or a father because the parent has passed away." There is a void, a feeling that there is a hole in their lives, despite the fact that they are still being given two parents' love.

There are other situations. For example, two parents may be married, but they either ignore the child because of their busy lives or one parent is too busy to offer the care and love required.

Children as they develop will concentrate mostly on their own emotions and desires. Young children are not developed enough mentally to understand there is more in the world than just what is before them or what they think about. To a child when a parent is missing, the first thought is "what have I done wrong." It is not that the parent is doing something wrong, but what have they done to make their parent absent.

You don't want your child to have these feelings. Whether you are a single parent or in a marriage, you want to protect your child from feeling there is a hole or loss in their life that is due to them.

For this reason, no matter the relationship or marriage situation you have, it is very important to have a healthy one that consistently offers stability.

Here are the reasons that people have children:

- They think their marriage will be stronger.
- They feel something is missing from their life and try to fill a hole.
- One person is trying to keep the other in the relationship, despite there is not enough love.
- An unplanned pregnancy occurs.
- Both parents are ready to accept a child in their life.
- A person wishes to have a child to share their love and raise a child who is genetically related.

Some of these reasons to have children are not valid. They set up a situation for the child to feel neglected or that something is missing. When both parents or two people in a relationship are ready to have a child, it is because they are in a place in their relationship that already provides stability. A person who is emotionally and financially prepared can also raise a child with love and affection. It is when you are not ready for a child in your life or when two parents are not on the same page that things can be difficult. It is not impossible, but you can end up hurting your children unintentionally when there is not stability in your marriage or relationship.

It does not mean you have to give up the idea of having a child. However, it is better to be prepared and ready in your life before you bring a child into the world. There are always possibilities of your child becoming hurt due to a failed marriage, even if your relationship and marriage are strong when you plan to have a child. There are also possibilities that you can hurt your child as you raise them by doing or saying the wrong thing.

For some children, simply speaking about an older sibling, always in front of them and ignoring what the child feels is most important, can leave a scar. It is a worry with no answer; however, if you set yourself up for a better situation and more stability before bringing a child into this world you have better odds.

There is no secret handbook or guide to raising children, but your true intentions and maturity will be felt.

YOUR RELATIONSHIP WITH YOUR PARTNER

Before you have a child, it is better for your relationship with your partner to be stable. Yes, things may happen later on, but this is not going to dwell on that. For now, your focus needs to be on whether or not, you and your partner are ready to bring a child into your family.

It is about the psychological preparedness you have gone through to accept a child in your life. No book can probably tell you just how much your life is going to change after your child arrives and for the rest of your life. Your children are going to need you and be involved in your life. Your marriage is not going to go back to what it once was pre-children.

You will need to accept that life after children will be forever changed.

You also have to be in a place in your life that is mature and ready to share the love you have for a child versus the desire to have a child because it is the next step in your marriage. There is a difference and both parents have to be on the same page.

Let's discuss pre-children for a moment. The first year of marriage is often a honeymoon stage, as well as questioning whether you made the right choice. You find out more about the person and life begins to find a routine.

You and your partner may have two or three date nights, where you go out, drink, meet friends, and have a good time. When you have children, you will find yourself lucky to get a babysitter so you can have one night in a month. Rather than you and your partner focusing on each other, there will be a new focus on your child's need. They will come first.

One parent can be better at accepting this than another. It can also be about emotional maturity. Is one parent still more interested in going out, playing video games, and travelling? Perhaps one of you is still in college and needs to focus all your time on studying, not raising a child? These are very important factors in your current relationship that can strain or influence how you form a relationship or bond with a child.

Your relationship has to be able to accept that it is the right time to have a child, emotionally.

- You should be at a maturity level where you can put your child's needs first, at all times.
- Your maturity needs to show that you are capable of being the parent.
- You also require proper communication with your partner to avoid some of the immature or angry arguments that can arise. Yes, arguments will

happen when two people are in close quarters, tired, and stressed. However, there is a difference in an argument because you are tired and because the other parent refuses to listen or provide consistency in parenting.

- Your maturity and ability to be a parent is about consistency and stability, where both parents agree on how to raise the child and compromise on certain issues.

Basically, your relationship needs to be on the same page, where you both want children, are both ready for the commitment, and you are both emotionally mature and prepared for the responsibility of parenting. As long as you can accept that your life will never be the same once you have a child and that they are your responsibility before anything else, then you should be ready to have a child.

You will not understand how much you are going to love your child, until you are holding your child in your arms. You can think about it and still not come close to the sudden epiphany you have when a child has arrived. It can change your perspective immediately, but for some who have yet to reach an emotional maturity, where "I" is still the first thing that pops into their head it may not change your perspective enough.

DO YOU HAVE...

A marriage, partnership, or are you single? It is rather helpful to view the different types of relationships a person might be in, as a way to examine the pros and cons. It can also help get you thinking about whether your relationship is as steady and stable as you think it is.

MARRIAGE

Being married is considered the most stable relationship you can be in. It is one where you have committed to another person for life, for better or worse. As we all know, marriage is not always stable. Things can be hidden or your acceptance of another's traits can change.

The pros of marriage are that you can show your baby and thus your child a committed relationship, one where you compromise and love each other, even thru the arguments you might have.

The cons of marriage are that you can find out things about your partner that you didn't know, as well as show your child how easy it is to break vows you made. Marriage can also be used as a weapon, where one refuses to divorce because of their vows and keeps a person in their child's life that may not be best for their child. Marriage can also be expensive to end should there be a cause.

PARTNERSHIP

A partnership is one with commitment, but without any paperwork to legally back it up. For some, there is always the feeling that you can leave when things go bad and for others there is no need to legally show a commitment you intend to keep for life. From the outside looking in a con can be that you are not showing your children how to make a commitment for life, but how to leave an escape hatch in any situation. On the other hand, without legally binding yourself to another, there are no messy divorce and court proceedings. You can still have a battle over child custody, should something go wrong.

SINGLE PARENTING

You may decide to have a child without a father. It is something that is more common with the scientific ability to fertilize eggs with a sperm donation. This route requires you to fill both positions as father and mother. It also means you only have a single income to depend on and your child may feel a loss because they do not have a father at all like other children.

However, you are also able to fill both roles, with your ideas on how to raise a child, without the conflict and compromise that can come along with being in a relationship.

Here are some questions to ask yourself about relationships and marriage:

- Are you in the first or second year of marriage?
- How often do you fight?
- If you fight, what are those fights about? Are they petty, filled with jealousy, or about important issues?
- Are there certain things you both disagree on?
- Is one of you ready for a child, but the other says "let's wait a little longer?"
- Are you ready to have someone else to focus on or do you still imagine a life of eating out, going to parties, or having fun with just the two of you?
- Do you include your family, or do you still have a feeling that you wish it to be just the two of you? Or does your partner?

If you still want holidays to be just the two of you or your partner does, then you are not ready to have a baby. If you fight often about the little things and have poor communication, then you are not ready.

CHAPTER 2: COMMUNICATION

Communication is part of a marriage and relationship, but it deserves its own chapter. Communication is one of the areas in life many of us have trouble with. A case and point: a sister was teasing her older brother, while helping him through a difficult divorce. Sensitive because of years of improper communication with the ex-wife, he justified his statement totally missing that his sister was teasing him. He admitted that sometimes he forgets that he has a level headed adult who is willing to help in all areas such as unloading things from the vehicle after a shopping trip versus someone who never even thought to help or think outside of her wants. So even people who understand each other quite well can find it difficult to communicate at times because of missed verbal or body language cues.

To help you develop better communication here are some tips:

- Listen, don't just hear. People will say all the time, "I'm listening," but if you ask them what was said or to repeat it verbatim there are usually words missing or the paraphrasing misconstrues the point. Listening is much different than just hearing. Listening is where the mind is engaged in memorizing what is being said in order to be exact and to discern the context of the words. Visual cues can be helpful in remembering a conversation.

For instance, an adult remembers a conversation she had with her dad at eight years old. It was a conversation she didn't fully understand because it was about politics and an upcoming election. However, she remembers why her father said he was tempted to vote, when he never found someone worth voting for in the election. She remembers the name of the person he thought was worth voting for and where and when the conversation happened. All she has to picture is the truck they were riding in.

If you do have trouble listening and understanding the context of the conversation, then you might want to try visual cues. Usually if you can picture one thing in your mind that helps you remember a few words, then you can get the rest of the words and digest the information.

- Don't analyze right away. One of the worst things you can do is immediately want to break into the conversation with your response or come up with a response that you dwell on. By thinking in your mind about what you want to say, you can miss a lot of what the other person is trying to tell you. It is better to listen to the person, if need be, ask questions, and then request a few moments to think about your response.
- Use patience. Some people are born with natural patience and others have to develop it. If you can write down your response, so you don't forget it and then go back to

listening to the person, you may find that you have the patience to listen better. It is when you are impatient to respond that you stop listening and thus you lose the importance of what the other person is trying to say.

- If necessary, start to develop methods that will help you gain more patience. Outside of your marriage, put yourself in situations where you need to be understanding, and patient to avoid creating a catastrophe. If you can learn it with others, you may find your communication is better in your marriage.

There is nothing wrong with enrolling in a communication course for married couples. You may need to research the one that will best fit your needs, but there are courses out there that help you learn how to listen, be patient, and respond in better ways when communicating.

Communication is often about emotions. Our emotions rise higher and suddenly we have misconstrued something or made a statement that was not our intention. When emotions run high, it is more difficult to find words in our memory that are right to express what we wish to say. By working on your communication, you can have a better marriage or relationship with your spouse, partner, or anyone else you are friends or related to.

CHAPTER 3:
OTHER RELATIONSHIPS IN YOUR LIFE

Along with changing your perspective in your married life, you will also need to look at other relationships you have in your life. Your child is going to be around your friends, family, and other people. Who they are exposed to during their life can drastically affect what they learn and their attitude as they grow up. This is not to say you want to shelter your child, but you do want to surround your child with those who are capable of showing proper love, affection, manners, and behaviors.

You will also find your relationships changing. Single friends who consistently go out and want you to go with them, are less of a priority. You may also find you no longer have a lot to talk about with them or you are too busy to do so. If your single friends like kids and enjoy hanging out with you in a family setting that is great, but a lot of the times the parents you meet in birthing classes or friends who are also having children are the people you will start to hang out with.

It is a chance for all of you to swap baby stories, such as my child is teething, or just took his/her first steps towards crawling. A lot of new parents also have a change of heart about how much help they are willing to accept from family.

Mature parents realize their parents have been through raising children and often figure their parents did things right or wrong depending on their relationship with them. This can matter when seeking advice. Most new parents actually see that their parents tried their best, when they are suddenly faced with a crying baby or a child that is not listening.

The point—the relationships you allow to form around you will have an impact on your children as they age. You want loving, doting people who will be a good example and not people who provide a poor example of behavior and manners.

An example of an incorrect choice: A young mother with two children needed to hire a babysitter, so she could return to work. She chose a person that seemingly had experience, an older person. This older person left the youngest child to play on her own, never held her, gave her attention, and basically just made sure both kids were fed and their bathroom needs were taken care of. She was of the school of belief that you can spoil a child with any attention, such as hugs, and play interaction. The babysitter's thoughts were, the child has to learn to do things on her own, even if it is to play a game by herself. The young mother was appalled. For a child to learn, she recognized that interaction is a good thing. Even if the interaction is based on socialization and learning, it is better than a child being ignored or in her opinion neglected by the babysitter.

Another example: Two divorced parents, where one parent has a new relationship, and the children are interacting with the new person. It was mentioned to the parent that sometimes the new person plays too rough. The reaction: "you (meaning the child) need to tell this person that the play is too rough." The parent didn't say "I'll speak with this new person in our lives," but rather told the child to say it. Yes, on the one hand it is good to teach a child to speak up, but on the other hand, if a new person in their lives is playing too rough, then it needs to be addressed by the parent if for nothing other than safety purposes.

Any person in your child's life that does not offer good manners, politeness in all situations, and appropriate behavior should not be around your child or there should be limited contact. This is especially important for babies and children who have yet to reach a developmental stage where they can differentiate good from bad, funny from too much, and the like.

There are certain people you will not want to cut relationships with. For example, family members are members you want your children to know, but you may not want a lot of time spent with those family members. It all has to do with the behavior and the amount of influence you want the person to have.

A family member capable of saying "I love you," have a hug, and "what did you do today or what fun things do you like to do," is better than one that yells, screams, or ignores the child.

For instance, what if your child has a grandmother who is depressed, puts down their child, and tries to enforce their "acceptable" thoughts on your child? Would you want your child around such an influence? Here is a true story:

A young boy was doing his chores as he was told. The grandmother did not think it proper for him to leave the other chores to his sister. The chore list and whose week it was to do these chores was listed on the fridge. The boy said he would follow what his parents' request of him and that his sister would do her chores while he did his. He was slapped for saying it and trying to follow his parents' request.

An influence like the grandmother was in some ways not good, but in others he was old enough to understand that the grandmother was not a very nice person, and while she should be respected as an elder did not usurp the rules of his household.

As you form relationships with adults, introduce your children to friends, family, and people in the school system, you want to determine which relationships may need to be monitored and others that are good for your child.

Babies are not yet capable of seeing behavior and understanding it completely. They do not know right from wrong, but keeping people in your life that will cause you stress will not help you raise a happy child. Your baby needs to be kept from seeing negative emotions, whenever possible.

CHAPTER 4: FINANCES

Relationships are one of the most important aspects to raising a happy, healthy baby. In fact, time has shown us that the love, affection, and proper behavior we teach our children is better than neglect and money. A child needs nurturing more than they need every item on the planet money can buy. Despite the need for more nurturing than cash, it is still in your best interest to focus on finances as you consider having a child.

According to an article in the Huffington Post from 2014, the middle income family will spend approximately $245,300 on their child from the time the child is born till they reach 18 years of age. This is for a child born in 2013 and is 1.8 percent higher than the projection from 2012, as it accounts for inflation. Most middle income families spend about $12,000 to $14,000 on their children per year.

The amount spent on a child in a year is a car, fully paid, and the amount spent on a child for 18 years is a decent home in some cities and towns. If you put these numbers in perspective, and realize that the number will increase as the inflation rate increases, then you could spend over $300,000 just raising your child for 18 years if your child is born in the next few years and more than that if you wait five to ten years.

Financial planning to raise a child needs to start before you are emotionally ready to have the child, to ensure that you are financially prepared when your first born child arrives.

Here is a breakdown of what you will require during pregnancy:

- Health insurance
- Income spent on making a will and power of attorney
- Income spent on a life insurance policy
- Medical expenses based on what your health insurance will or will not pay for maternity fees
- Income spent on creating a nursery and getting the essentials for taking care of your newborn
- Extra savings in the event of a difficult, high risk pregnancy or birth complications
- Income for buying new clothing and other essentials as your baby grows

During the first year, you will need multiple outfits per day, the income to pay for washing these clothes, as well as income to buy new outfits as your child grows. A newborn can already be born out of the newborn clothing sizes. In a month, your child may be wearing outfits for a 3 month or 6-month old. The point is you may need to buy new clothes, sell the old ones, and ensure that you have the finances to handle the quick growth rate of your baby.

As your child reaches a year, you will want to have different stimulating toys and activities for your child. Each year, your baby will need new clothing, new care items, and new toys to help them develop their brains and gain an education, and proper behavior.

Once school starts, expenses will increase as you buy school supplies, new outfits for school, and much more relating to school needs.

If your finances are wiped out before you have a maternity bill, it will make things difficult. You may not be able to provide even the basic items your newborn needs for their arrival and the years after.

Here is a list of things you may want to consider as you do a little financial planning:

- Housing
- Food
- Transportation
- Healthcare
- Childcare/education
- Clothing
- Miscellaneous
- Emergency

These topics are usually expenses related to your new baby, but you can also take it a step further and list all your expenses and income. As you do with any budget, you will want to have a list of what you make, what your projected expenses will be, and what you already have in savings.

Smart parents are those who begin to add to their emergency fund the minute they find out they are pregnant. These same financially intelligent individuals shop around, determine what they need to spend for the safety and comfort of their children, and create a budget of what will be spent.

Remember, you can always sell the clothing that no longer fits or the items your child no longer needs, as long as safety permits. However, you will not be able to recoup all the losses and you may wish to keep some things for a second child.

You can also realize that spending $2 on a onesie outfit is better than spending $10 or more. Your child is going to grow out of their clothing quickly. There is no need to spend more than you can afford or should spend to be reasonable.

You are going to want to take time off from work to spend with your baby, to bond, and you don't want to have stress due to financial worries. There are also things you will want to do with your child as they age. For example, when your children are tall enough to ride all the rides at Disney World or Land, you will want to take them there. You may have local zoos, museums, and local, national sites that are important, which you will want to take your child to. It is all about being able to afford all of this that will make you want to start setting up a fund for your child now, before they are even a tiny strawberry size in your belly.

WILLS AND LIFE INSURANCE

These two items may not make a lot of sense to you right now, for why it must happen before pregnancy or when you find out you are pregnant. The fact is, if you are 18 or older, you should already have a will and a life insurance policy. The life insurance policy needs to be in place to cover your funeral costs and any debt you may have. The will tells how any savings you have that is not used for paying debts should be divided up. A person without a will who dies may leave their partner without enough cash flow to survive for the time period the estate is in probate. Any household without a will automatically enters probate.

There is no reason to create more stress should something happen. Furthermore, your will and life insurance need to outline a guardian in the event one or both parents are killed or hurt. Accidents and unforeseen events occur, but you can plan financially for these situations. A part of financial matters is to pay for your wills and life insurance to avoid added stress, particularly when there is a life depending on you.

Above all else, when it comes to your baby or the thought of a baby in the near future, you do not need to add to your stress and concerns by forgetting to be ready. These negatives will impact your relationship with your child. Your baby may not understand the word "stress," but they will feel it in you. A happy baby is raised when you are happy, and not worried or stressed.

DOING THE THINGS, YOU LOVE

You have dreams. You might have already created a bucket list of things you wish to do before you die. Life is uncertain, which can make it hard for you to fulfill your list. Since you are reading this book, you obviously wish to become a parent. But what about some of the other things you hope to do?

There was a couple, married for 42 years. Before children, they went to Hawaii, toured Europe for a month, and traveled around the USA. After children, they took road trips around the lower 48, a cruise to Mexico with their kids, and were able to see two grandchildren born. The one thing both of them agreed on was to travel certain places before children because they didn't want to be too old later on. They saw a lot of older couples taking European trips that could barely enjoy everything because of physical restrictions. Some couples on their trip had food limitations, others had physical limits because of knee surgeries, and health problems. When they came back from their trip, the couple was happy and more ready to have children. It also turns out that it was the best move they could have made because the husband developed early onset dementia and passed away before his 64th birthday.

Now, you might look at this lesson and say, "Gosh, I'd better have children today, just in case," but that is not the point. The actual point is that you shouldn't have regrets in any part of your life, whether it is in doing things together as a married couple, having children, or getting your finances all set before you have children.

This section is asking that you take some of the money you have and decide how you want to use it, to avoid having any regrets in life, whether it is about travel, raising your children with better than you had, or anything else.

CHAPTER 5: EMOTIONS

Emotional readiness is just one part of the entire concept of "emotions." Your relationship and how you interact with your partner certainly matters. Yet, there is a slew of emotions, you arc going to feel as you work towards getting pregnant, are pregnant and then have your baby. You are not always going to be happy. You won't want to show happiness 100 percent of the time, and yet, your baby needs to feel love, happiness, and reassurance—not conflict. How you approach your desire to have children and after having a baby will determine whether you are always stressed or not.

One of the things that is important for soon-to-be-parents is to gain mindfulness before you have your child. Mindfulness can help you with the variety of emotions you are going to experience. Before getting into the "how," it will be best to discuss some of the emotions you will start to feel.

Before you hear the words, "You are pregnant," you will start to have several emotions. For some couples, there are obstacles. It may be related to stress or to health conditions. A person with thyroid problems may have trouble getting pregnant and then be a high risk pregnancy. More often than you may also be aware, the first pregnancy for a lot of women ends in a miscarriage in the first trimester. One reason for a first pregnancy miscarriage is a misaligning of the genes to form a healthy, viable fetus.

You will need to prepare yourself for the possibility of a miscarriage or even a stillbirth. These are not things you want to think about as happening, but it can still happen even with the best advancements in medicine that we have today. A loss is always going to be a loss. How you are able to get passed the loss is going to matter for your next attempt at having a child.

There are also numerous families that have to seek help for the fertilization process. You may begin to obsess about taking your temperature, monitoring your menstrual cycle, and try to have intercourse at the perfect time for a pregnancy to occur.

For others, it is easier to be laid back, to stop birth control, and allow nature to take its course. Studies have found that when your emotions are high, raw, and overstressed it is harder to become pregnant. Women who do not have regular menstrual cycles due to stress may take years to become pregnant because stress can stop ovulation.

When you wish to have a child, you have to be in an emotional state that will be best for you to get pregnant, as well as continue to have a good emotional state that will help you raise a happy baby. Of course, one can say that you need to have controlled emotions, but it doesn't mean you can change who you are deep down and how you react to your emotions, without trying.

Your best option is to learn mindfulness or other techniques that you are willing to follow as a way to reduce your stress and gain an emotional stability that will help you get pregnant, get through the pregnancy, and face the changes in your life that come with a newborn child.

MINDFULNESS

Mindfulness is a state of conscious awareness of "something." In this case, it will be your emotions and the emotions of your partner or spouse. You are trying to achieve a state where you can accept your emotions and other's to reduce your stress, feel happier, and enjoy the new path you are about to embark on.

1. What is your will? Obviously, it is to have a child. However, in this chapter it is also to reduce your anxious emotions and replace them with happy, ready emotions to accept a child in your life. You have to start with determining a mindfulness goal that will alleviate your anxiety.

2. Open your mind to see things from a different perspective. Let's say, you are having trouble getting pregnant. You have tried the natural way and your medical history shows no problems in conceiving. Is

there a different way you can look at conceiving to reduce your stress and concern that you will never have a child to love? Perhaps, you are more stressed because you are trying to have a child when you are extremely busy on a project at work, and all you need is a vacation for the miracle to happen.

3. Patience is a word you will often hear in conjunction with being mindful. Patience is a quality you need to work on in order to challenge the anxiety you have. You will be more anxious if you keep dwelling on what has not happened. Consider thinking, "when the time is right, when destiny, fate, or whatever aligns, then you will have a child."

4. Acknowledgement is necessary as a part of understanding your experiences and what is currently happening. There may be no reason for you to have trouble conceiving, but the reality is that you are stressed, busy, or simply desiring a child too much to relax for nature to provide what you wish to have. Take a step back and accept the reality of now, and discover what you might be able to change.

5. Striving towards your goals because of a high desire can actually hinder you. Mindfulness teaches you to be non-striving. You don't have to cling, to reject, or to live in the future. Rather enjoy the now as a way to reduce an anxiety you might feel.

If you need to use a journal to help you reduce your stress and be more mindful of your feelings and that of your partner/spouse.

TYPICAL EMOTIONS AFTER BIRTH

You will want to draw again on mindfulness after your child is born. You will have plenty of emotions, including a wealth of love that rises in your heart. New parents are often tired, worried, and stressed. They turn to more experienced mothers and start to ask questions over every little thing. When you are stressed in front of your baby, they will feel it. If you start to cry, yell, or speak your frustration, your baby is bound to smile less, feel crankier, and want to cling to you more.

Here are a few things that can help with after your baby arrives:

- Have an hour to yourself, where you read a book, sleep, or take a bath. During this time, your spouse is going to take charge of your baby's needs.
- You will also give your spouse this same amount of time.
- Ask a family member or friend to babysit for one hour, even in the first three months. It is hard. You don't want to miss anything and you feel like you cannot leave, but leave. You'll be saner if you do. You just need an hour with your partner or spouse.

- Do not consider work as a getaway. Work has just as many stressors that can affect your emotions. Instead, of running away to work and feeling like you have a break from your child, you'll come back tired from work. If you work at home, then it will make it more difficult for you to feel as though you have gotten away.

You do not have to have time each day, although it is best if you can have an hour with your spouse/partner, and an hour to yourself each day. Strive for at least one time a week, where you both have an hour alone and an hour together with just each other.

ALWAYS PLAN A TIME FOR YOURSELF

Whether you have had a child or not, it is important for you to have time to yourself at least once a week. Yes, it is great to spend all your time with your spouse or partner, but you can still get tired of the other person. Your marriage can become stronger if you have at least an hour to yourself to relax. Being away from the person while each of you at work is not enough even before children. It also does not mean to go out and spend time in a noisy place with friends. You also need to do that, but what it means to have a time to yourself means that you are alone. You are with yourself, analyzing your emotions, thoughts, and desires. You are just "existing" without the pressure of entertaining someone else or taking care of another.

CHAPTER 6: TIMING

Timing or time is not about the stages of pregnancy or the time it might take to get pregnant. Rather, in this section is it about timing the attempt to have a child, as well as the amount of time you will spend with your child.

First, you want to check your emotions and your maturity level. Yes, this is a statement you have already seen, but one that must be repeated with regards to timing. Your maturity level will determine if you are truly ready to have a child and to deal with the changes that will occur after you have a baby. If you already need to have time to yourself and cannot see your spouse/partner's needs first, then you still need time to mature.

When you can put other people ahead of your wants and desires, you are ready to have a child. Now, you have to ask is your partner/spouse in the same place. Is your spouse putting you first all the time and not trying to take care of themselves? Is your spouse too self-involved? Perhaps you or your spouse have a job that takes all your time and you cannot focus on a new addition to your family? These are the questions and things you need to assess as you consider the timing of having a child.

If your marriage or relationship is rocky or filled with a lot of stress due to work, finances, or other concerns, then the timing may not be right to try and conceive.

Most importantly, when considering timing is the acceptance that your child is going to require all of your time before you will have time for yourself.

Children need you to spend as much time as possible with them. A newborn baby will need a routine where you have feedings, naps, bath time, and fulfill other care needs. Meeting the minimum needs of your child is not enough. Yes, anyone can feed a baby, change their diaper, and provide a bath.

Your baby needs to feel loved and secure. This is not done just by seeing to their needs. It is done by holding your child, interacting with them, even though they may not understand everything. At night, when you want to watch a favorite TV show, you can sit in your favorite spot, watch TV, and hold your baby. Letting your baby grab your finger or your shirt, while you watch the show is just another way to ensure you are interacting.

At various times of the day or evening after work, making faces, noises, or holding your baby will also be a way to show them they are loved and safe. It is your interactions, when you are happy and relaxed that will help the most in terms of raising a happy, healthy baby into a healthy, happy toddler, child, teenager, and adult.

For some parents, they do not realize the time they spend with their baby is as important as when their child is able to interact more. Yes, they understand a bond is formed, but after a few months it can seem less important to interact. It is still extremely important to interact, provide hugs, and there is nothing that is "spoiling" the child by offering consistent, constant, attention. Spoiling occurs when a child is always the center of attention, they can do nothing wrong, and are given everything they ever ask for. Providing attention, love and a secure feeling, is being a good parent.

Let's say you walk in the door, say hello, give your baby a hug and a kiss, and then you disappear into a room for the rest of the evening. Is this good parenting or bad?

What if you walk in the door, say hello, provide a hug and a kiss, spend 30 minutes with your baby interacting with their toys, making faces, having a meal with them, and putting them to bed. Is this good parenting or bad?

You probably said the second example is a better form of parenting because there is interaction, versus parenting where the person acts like they care, but instead goes into a different room and doesn't come out except perhaps to grab a plate of food.

If the first words out of your mouth are, "hi, missed you, I need to get work done," then there is something wrong. Your baby, who will continue to grow and age, needs attention, will seek it, and will want to cling more to the parent who is not providing it, in hopes their love will be seen. It is this point that makes time important not only in when to have a child, but also in being able to give your child the time they need with you to be happy and well adjusted.

CHAPTER 7: PREGNANCY

Several factors can be discussed about pregnancy. Entire books are made just on the pregnancy stage alone. Many of the books tell you what to expect while you are pregnant. They explore how your body is going to change, how to deal with the emotions and the changes, as well as the miracle that you are undergoing carrying a child. This section is not a short explanation of all the stages of pregnancy. It is not about what to expect or even what your child needs in the few months of their life. It is going to discuss salient points that can determine if you are at a point in your life to be ready for a pregnancy and a few tips.

When you or your spouse becomes pregnant, there are certainly physical changes. You both will notice the physical changes, feel an emotional pull that there is a baby growing inside its mother. Many parents begin to feel excitement and love for the child. There are some parents who need to hold their child for the first time before a true emotional connection is made. It does not mean you are going to be a bad parent, if the reality of a child has not hit you until that baby is in your arms. It just means it takes you a little longer to accept that your reality is changing and there is someone else to love.

There are definitely emotional changes based on the mother's hormones. Crying, laughing, anger, and many other emotions can be felt. It is natural, and again something many other books go into.

As previously stated, a miscarriage can be a factor. Try as you might to prepare for something going wrong in your pregnancy, there really is no way to prepare. But, you can move on from it. You can gain strength from a loss and try to believe that there is another reason for why you have to wait a little longer to have a baby to hold.

More importantly, you do not have to wait to have a happy baby in your arms. When you are pregnant, this is when you start to help your baby to be happy. Yes, on a mental level they do not know what this means, but you do. You know whether you are stressed, overworking, or taking the time to pay attention to the miracle that you are growing inside of you.

Studies show that a baby in the womb develops better, as well as having more intelligence as a growing child, if classical or relaxing music is played during pregnancy. If the mother relaxes, versus keeps stressing over many things, a baby is happier in their life. Your baby can feel, even if there is no consciousness or understanding. There are instinctual feelings your baby has.

When you are pregnant, you need to reduce your stress as much as possible. A part of this is being ready to have a child in all aspects of your life.

Yes, you have to be prepared if there are medical issues. You may need to change your life if you have a high risk pregnancy. You also need to accept a possible loss if you have a medical issue or a high risk pregnancy. But, remember you have mindfulness to get you through the tough emotions. You also have a husband or partner to help you through the difficulty. It is when you forget that you are creating a part of each of you with a new life and that you are supposed to be there for each other that you can increase your stress, feel alone, and even depressed.

One thing you might try is setting up the nursery together. Make it an activity that shows how much you are both looking forward to your child, as well as gaining an understanding of how your life is about to change.

Your happy voices, talks, and interactions, while the baby is in the womb can help bring a happy baby into your life.

There is one tip that all parents need to know—sometimes babies just cry. It does not mean they are unhappy or that something is terribly wrong. In fact, babies cry to get exercise, especially, when they are too young yet to crawl or move a great deal. You will begin to learn the differences between upset, needing something, and exercise cries.

As long as you are happy, without stress, and communicating prior to pregnancy, during the pregnancy, and especially after the birth, your child will be happy from the womb

.

Chapter 8: The Caregiver Rule

The caregiver role is one you are going to fill as a parent to your child. There is a rule among caregivers that if you cannot take care of yourself first, then you will not be able to take care of someone else. It is because you have to be in a healthy situation both physically and emotionally in order to handle taking care of someone else who is going to demand your time.

You might think this does not apply to you. You may be thinking that you are having a child, someone who will need your love and someone you will want to take care of all the time.

However, the truth is much different. You will not be able to take care of them all the time. Your child is going to need you 24/7, in fact, you will wish you had another full day of time in a day just to do everything you need to do and take care of your child. As you spend more time focusing on someone else, you are going to stop looking at yourself and taking care of you.

Yes, in one part you do need to focus on your child. Keep your relationship good with your partner, but you also need to focus on yourself in a type of routine. It is more than taking an hour each day or week after your first have your child. It is about keeping some of the things in your life that you love.

You'll want to sacrifice certain things in your life. At first, you might say you don't need to read for now, you can always pick up a book a little later when your child is older. Unfortunately, it is very easy to leave behind a cycle and never go back to it.

You will start to miss the things you once loved. You'll even become bitter that you are unable to do some of the things you have always loved. It is not a happy situation to be in.

There is a way to ensure that this does not happen. Do not give up the things you love, completely. Yes, your life will change. Yes, it will be a little harder for you to do everything you once loved, but there are ways for you to keep doing some of what you like.

Pick one hobby. What hobby do you love the most? What can you feel comfortable still doing? Even if it is reading a book in the bath, there are ways to keep your hobbies going.

The trouble is, most of us think about having a child, realize the focus has to be on their needs and providing proper attention, and forget what we once loved until we become too bitter or tired.

You do not want to enter into the caregiver cycle, where you forget to do things for yourself and instead focus all of your love and attention on the person who needs it most. Yes, to a point the other person is your main focus, but you cannot lose sight of who you truly are either.

Here is an example:

A person is constantly catching colds because they forget to take their vitamins, forget to eat proper meals, and is always preparing meals, baths, play time for their child. Do you think always have a cold is doing the child any good? Of course, you cannot let yourself become run down, tired, or cranky because your child will see this. They will feel it and wonder what is wrong.

It is far better to set aside time for the basic things, including some time to enjoy a hobby or reflect on who you are. As a mother or father, you are going to find yourself evolving and changing. Who you were pre-child is not who you are going to be once the baby is born. So make certain to follow the caregiver rule—physically and emotionally take care of yourself by keeping at least one hobby that helps you exercise, remember who you are, or simply allows you to relax when you need to. Relax and recharge—these two words should repeat through your mind, to help you keep them fresh in your mind.

CHAPTER 9: DISCIPLINE—THE RULES

It is best for you to decide some topics before you even have a baby to look after, let alone a child in need of discipline. Establishing the rules prior to having a child, helps you see what both you and your partner feel regarding certain "hot" topics. Discipline is just one subject that parents can be in disagreement over. Other subjects you might disagree on include religion, politics, parental influence, people in your life, and even what baby food brand to buy.

Have you ever had a talk with your partner or spouse on the above topics? If you have not, then you need to do so now before a pregnancy. If you are unable to agree on how to raise a child, particularly on some of the most important issues, then you are not ready to bring a new life into your world.

Yes, to a degree there are decisions you can make as they arise. For example, which preschool is your child going to go to? The decision about preschool is something to decide when your child is closer to the age to enter a program. Some of your decisions will need to be generalizations.

- You both agree your child needs to go to preschool.
- You both agree that when it is time for discipline, you will each discipline your child, with the same methods, and at the time of the incident. One parent raised his child, stating, "my mother always said 'wait till your

dad gets home,' I'd always forget what I'd done by then and later it was a statement to fear." This parent believed in disciplining in the moment so that less fear, and more understanding could be reached.

- You both agree to choose food that is natural, without preservatives or artificial flavors.

The list and suggestions can go on and on. The point is that you should both agree because it is in the best interest of the child. If you do not discuss these points and at least agree on the generalizations, then you are leaving yourselves open to fights later on when it is important to be happy and less stressed in front of your child.

You can also leave your child open to confusion. For example, what happens if one parent does not follow through on discipline. They might say, "if you do not eat, then you are not going to get any food later when you are hungry," but then the parent gives in and allows the child to have a snack. How likely is it that the child is going to believe the words and not repeat the same refusal to eat again and again? If the child gets away with it once, then they will try to get away with it again and again. You want to start out without any room for "getting away" with something that is against your rules.

A common phrase a mom or dad used to ask a child, "did you ask your dad/mom if you could?" In other words, did you already ask one parent and were told no, so you are now asking to see if the other parent will allow something? If parents are on the same page with discipline and all topics, then it is easy to see through the child's "devious" behavior and gain the truth. It is also a perfect time for a lesson. You can state if you already asked one parent, then you know the answer and in asking me, you are still going to get the same answer. If the child tries to lie, it opens an opportunity to catch them in the lie and stop such behavior before it starts.

From these examples, you can recognize, why you want to have a general sense of how you both think and what you both agree on raising your child. If you already cannot agree, fight about these topics like discipline, then you have to either compromise or admit that until you can compromise you should not have a child.

If your life is going to be full of arguments or frustrations before children, it will only continue when you have another person to take care of.

CHAPTER 10: HOUSING AND STABILITY

A lot of the focus has been on ensuring that you have everything prepared for your child, in a general way. You learned about relationships, financial matters, communication, pregnancy factors not in other books, and many other things. You might think that housing and stability should be a part of the finances and perhaps, the topic should be. However, I think it carries enough importance to be on its own.

Yes, it is a financial concept. You will need to have a home that you can provide your child and be able to afford. In fact, you have to have a home that ensures there is shelter for your growing baby. You have to factor in the cost of the housing payment or rent for each month. It is rather a common sense topic in that respect.

In terms of this section, there is something you need to think about even more than having a house and the payment you are going to make. It is about the ability to keep that home and ensure you can provide a stable home throughout your young child's life.

What if you were 8 years old and you moved four times, all in the same town? It is not like a child moving four times because their parent is changing jobs or in the military. It is a move due to instability of the finances to take on such a home.

When you are thinking about having a child, ask yourself this question:

Do I need multiple rooms, with multiple bathrooms, for three people? Do I need to spend $1,000 a month just to find a house that will be comfortable for the first eight years of my child's life?

We tend to go for huge homes with two or three thousand square feet, when the right house with 1,000 square feet will be enough. There are possibilities for you to upgrade your home size as your family increases, but the better thing to do is keep a house that you are not spending half of your monthly income on.

Let's say you only make $2,000 a month, and half of that is going to rent or a mortgage. Are you truly able to buy groceries, toys, and other things you and your child need? Chances are, you cannot. You probably use two or three credit cards to make it happen in this type of situation. There is no reason for you to be worried about your housing.

It is understandable that in some places rent or mortgages will be expensive. However, there are other solutions. You can have a longer drive to reduce your expenses or you can downsize the size of your home to get one that you can afford. The other option is to wait until you are financially solvent enough without children to purchase a home without a mortgage or a very small mortgage.

CHAPTER 11: WORK AND STABILITY

Along with home stability, where your child can grow up feeling safe and as if they do not have to move all the time, you want to consider work and stability before having a child. There is reality and there is hope.

The reality is that you may not have your current job forever. The hope is that you will. Families that learn they are going to have a child and start saving so they have at least six months to a year of all their expenses saved up by the time the child is born, can relax a little should something go wrong with their job. A family that lives month to month, without enough money to pay their expenses, let alone pay for an added child cannot afford to have their job disappear.

The mortgage crisis of 2008 should be a lesson for anyone who thinks that jobs are everlasting. People who did nothing, but chose to work for a company lost their jobs. They lost their jobs because the market turned, companies had to downsize, and it didn't matter that they could perform well in their current position. Raises were cut, insurance plans were reduced, and several families lost their homes. It is a lesson that nothing is ever absolute.

Yet, there are also signs that things are not going well in your current company or perhaps in your department. If you are more mindful, you will be able to recognize the signs of whether or not your job could be in jeopardy or if there are things you can do to help you gain more security in the working world.

The first is to start saving now, and wait to have a child. The second, is to have a second source of income that you can depend on if the economy or your company begins to have problems. Mainly, you want to be aware of what is happening on various levels in your company to know whether or not there is a long term, even a retirement option in that company for you.

Sometimes young parents think they will be in the same field forever, and yet they have a child, realize they have a capacity for a different type of job, and then decide to go back to school. It is okay to switch jobs or go back to school. However, you also need to have stability for the first several years you are raising your child. You cannot be worrying where your next paycheck will come from.

If you don't feel stability in your current job or you are unhappy, it is not the time to have a child. You should be confident in your choices and know that you are willing to be in your job, no matter how much you don't like it if the need is there. In other words, you may not be able to find another job because there is nothing available, thus you need to be ready to at least live with your choices. Your child needs stability not only in the money that is coming in, but your ability to cope when things are not perfect.

CONCLUSION

Thank you again for purchasing this book!

I hope this book was able to help you with your needs and to satisfy your reading pleasures.

Parenting is 80 percent hope that you will do something right and raise a healthy, happy child. There is no manual that can help you raise your baby, other than to tell you the stages of their development.

As a guide, this was designed to help you think about all the aspects of your life that will need to change once you bring a baby into this world. It is nothing more and nothing less.

You are ready to be a parent if you have already thought of much of the content that was in here or are able to reflect and say "that makes sense." Congratulations and enjoy raising your happy baby.

Finally, if you enjoyed this book, please take the time to share your thoughts and post a review on Amazon. It would be greatly appreciated!

Thank you and good luck!

PARENTING

ADVICE FOR NEW PARENTS ON RAISING A STRONG WILLED CHILD

BY HELEN WHITE

TABLE OF CONTENTS

Introduction...63

Chapter 1: Newborn Care and Nurturing............................65

Chapter 2: Guide for Dads in Dealing with Newborns..........71

Chapter 3: Newborn Development 78

Chapter 4: Newborn & Infant Nutrition 86

Chapter 5: Early Education for the Toddler 102

Chapter 6: Disciplining Toddlers 112

Conclusion 119

INTRODUCTION

Ah...Parenting, the ultimate long-term investment many married or unmarried couples make for various reasons. Would be parents; be prepared to put in far more than what you bargained for, at least for a particular time.

Parenting cultures all around the world have different variations of stress levels and often; the happiness of the couples themselves takes a dive because all the attention goes to the child. But, that is only if you aren't ready to be a parent, or you aren't doing it right.

However, ask any parent and they'll tell you that having a child is the most rewarding decision they've ever made. Parenting involves a lot of things, and it encompasses every aspect of a human being- emotions, feelings, and mental readiness and of course physical and time change.

Parents need to do everything for their infants until they are ready to spread their wings and fly, and this is from reading and talking and teaching their children to lead by example, making values and beliefs clear and sharp- parents have an enormous influence over their child's early developments. Of course, as the child grows and enters their first tastes of life, they are exposed to various other influences such as their teachers, classmates, the bus driver, the lunch operator and nanny even. No matter what the outside influences are, the child's first few lessons in life is a good start to ensure the child knows what is important and right and good.

For the parent, it is important to be aware that each and every child that comes into this world has their very own temperament and characteristics, and it is up the parent to provide a necessary boundary between the child and the world, in preparing them for independent living.

This book will explore various methods and ways as well as tips and tricks of parenting a child especially from the time of birth till the child is one or two years old. This book will also give a good overview of the development stages of a child as well as the range of nutrition that is essential for a growing baby.

CHAPTER 1:

NEWBORN CARE AND NURTURING

Having a newborn baby is one of the most exciting things in parents' lives! But no matter how much of research you do and how many moms you speak to before your little bundle arrives, you won't be truly prepared for the first few weeks of motherhood until you go through it on your own.

Sure you and your partner stock up the standard baby supplies like diapers and bodysuits, you baby proof your home, your set up a nursery, you read about nutrition and all that but essentially, newborn care isn't about the baby alone. It is also about the mother. Here're some tips on pre and post-delivery preparation that you can prepare for yourself and your newborn baby:

BEFORE YOUR NEWBORN ARRIVES

MEAL PREPPING

When the baby comes, you'll find yourself with little time for many things which includes cooking healthy meals. Unless you have the luxury of employing a nanny or housemaid to help you out, or a husband, cooking and eating at the right times can be an arduous task. For that reason, meal prepping ahead of time and freezing them can help you when you are hungry and need something nutritious to eat. Casseroles and lasagna, wraps and even soups freeze well. Make double batches of what you are cooking and put half of them away for a future meal. Ensure that your pantry is properly stocked with simple items that you can use to whip up a quick and healthy meal. This will come handy when you find yourself with sleepless nights. Also to have on hand are crackers, pasta and of course, cereal.

STOCK YOUR SUPPLIES

Before your baby arrives, make sure your home is stocked with the essentials such as food, water, clothing and toiletries because then you do not have to keep running to the store every time you run out of something. Grocery shopping after the baby arrives will be with the baby and never alone. This will also help your partner or husband- even he can spend more time with you and the baby instead of running errands and buying supplies. Not sure what to stack on? Here are some things to add to your list:

1. Formula and feeding bottles- the formula is necessary if you are not nursing but you may still need it to supplement even if you are breastfeeding.
2. Diapers- yes you will need loads of this- probably 10 to 12 for the first few weeks
3. Baby Wipes- Babies poop, pee, burp, puke, and spit- you are going to need loads of wipes for this

4. Tissues & Towels- again, because there's always something that needs to be wiped.

5. Cribs & Bassinets- It is always nice to have extra of these just to you can stretch out the time between doing the laundry

6. Baby bodysuits- the easiest to open for diaper changes and the easiest to 'suit up' your baby

7. Maternity pads- not something most women talk about but celebrities like Olivia Wilde and Chrissy Teigen have been talking about all the effects of post-pregnancy, and this includes maternity pads. You will need a supply of this for the next couple of weeks.

8. Nursing Pads- Your breasts will likely leak in between feedings, and this is pads will help prevent the leak from seeping into your clothes.

9. Stool Softener- something to have because some post-pregnancy medication that you take might make you slightly constipated. Check with your doctor on which stool softeners are safe to take while nursing. Try not to push when going to the bathroom because this will lead to hemorrhoids.

10. Protein bars- This is great to have not only when you are working out but also after you have given birth. It is perfect for snacking on days that you don't want to eat your frozen meals, or you are suddenly in need of something to munch on.

11. Diaper rash ointments-Brands such as Burt's Bees Baby Bee Diaper Ointment and Triple Paste and even Babyganics Diaper Rash Cream is great to have as they are super effective, and they are organic.

12. Antibacterial gel- Antibacterial gel is essential to keep for any reason especially when you need to get a quick diaper change done in places that do not have changing stations. Quickly dab on some gel on your hands to wash them and get to changing the diapers

WHEN THE NEWBORN ARRIVES HOME

TAKE TURNS FEEDING

Take turns to feed the baby because newborns have to eat at least every 3 to 4 hours. Whether it is the dad or a relative, take turns to feed the baby. If you are nursing, pump your breast milk into a bottle and save it for later by freezing it. Experts say that this is good to do after a few weeks of giving birth and to give your baby as much fresh breast milk as possible so that both mother and child get into the rhythm of breastfeeding before introducing the bottle. This is also done to encourage milk production and to avoid nipple confusion. Nursing is always easier than pumping as the milk is always ready in the breast and always at the right temperature.

ASK FOR HELP

Unfortunately, not all of us have a nanny or a baby nurse helping us when we get home from the hospital. But then again, that's what our spouses are for right? Even if you are a single mother, get help from a family member. When you are a new mother, any help is welcomed especially for the sleep-deprived mother. Having some time off to shower and put on some fresh clothes, taking a break or a nap will help you so much.

HANDLING THE NEWBORN

Some parents have a very natural ability with children probably because they have had some experience with newborns of family and friends. But even so, when you have your child to care for, the fragility of the newborn can be a pretty intimidating experience. When handling your newborn here are some basic things to remember:

- Wash your hands before handling your newborn-babies do not have very strong immune systems, so they are very susceptible to infections and germs. Make sure anyone handling your child is not sick and washes their hands. Keep yours clean too.
- Support the baby's neck and head- babies' bodies are fragile as their bones and muscles are not developed

yet. Always make sure to support their head and neck when carrying your baby or when laying them down.

- No rough play- this is pretty obvious, but again, babies are fragile so do not shake your newborn or do any sharp movements or even shaking. There are more subtle ways of dealing with a baby and if you do not know what it is, then go for parenting classes.

- Make sure your newborn is fastened correctly to the stroller, car seat or carrier. Also, do not leave your newborn in the car!

Chapter 2: Guide for Dads in Dealing with Newborns

The face of parenting is changing as more and more women become working mothers or even sole breadwinners of the family. Parenting in today's world is not only for the mother but the father as well because as traditional gender roles are blurred, and both sets of parents take equal share of responsibility of parenting the child. For the first-time dad, things change a lot for them too, and the excitement and exhaustion can be so overwhelming, and you'll find time moving so fast. As with mother's, here is a set of tips and advice for the first-time dads.

You are NOT the clueless husband/partner

Men also have gender stereotypes that are often not as vivid or spoken about as gender stereotypes for women. For men who become first-time fathers, they are often labeled as clueless or not interested as much in raising a child or more focused on the job than raising a family. Well, for millennial dads out there- break this stereotype! Show them what kind of father you can be and the husband or partner that you are for your other half. It takes two of you to make a child, so it takes the same equal responsibility of raising one. Do not become the clueless husband. Read up on parenting tips, how to help the new mother, what you can do to make your wife or partner well rested and how to bond with your child. Sign up for parenting classes if you have to. Remember that you aren't the only one who is new at this- your partner/spouse is new at this too.

HELP HER

Do not wait to be asked for help. Help at every possible point. Your wife or partner is probably as overwhelmed as you are with the new baby so your helping hand in this new chapter will benefit the both of you long-term. Your wife is probably too focused on whether she is doing things right or is afraid of getting things wrong. This is where you come in as both an emotional, mental and physical support for her. Jump in and help your wife because helping out without being asked will give her the confidence that you both are a team, and you are both in this together. If she's feeding the baby- then get the house organized- clean, mop, and cook or do the laundry. Take feeding time seriously and let your wife sleep or rest. Run errands to stock up on supplies, take her to visit the doctor for her checkup and appointments. There is so much you can do without her asking you for help.

BOND WITH YOUR BABY

There is no perfect time to bond with your child. That time is now. Yes, your wife is mothering the baby, but there are countless of times that you can create your fatherly bond with your child. Tell her to take a break and take this time to tend to the baby. There are many ways to bond with your child such as changing the baby's diapers, feeding the baby, playing with the baby or even just holding your newborn. The point is, the slightest tender touch of your hand is all the baby needs to start a bond. A connection is created between child and parent and when this happens, this connection will be permanently etched in their minds and strengthen the bond for years to come.

BOTH PARENTS WILL HAVE DIFFERENT PARENTING STYLES

And that is fine. Mothers and father have different ways of dealing with newborns and their older children. Think about how it was for you while you were growing up. Think about what your father did that was different from your mother's-various parent styles is what helps the child to grow up confident, responsible, reliable and believe in themselves. Neither parent should force the other to do it their way. Both parents should have the freedom in dealing with the baby as how comfortable they seem fit as long as it isn't wrong (like drugging the baby, so it sleeps).

JUST BECAUSE SHE'S THE MOTHER, THAT DOESN'T MAKE HER THE EXPERT

Probably one of the biggest misconceptions some new fathers have is that they think new mothers know it all. Being a mother takes trial and error and so does being a father. No matter how many kids you have, you will still learn new things because guess what- each child you bring into this world has their characteristics which you need to deal with in a different way.

Don't Make her Feel Bad

New mothers are bound to forget things or are not on point when it comes to certain things at home or she may not be groomed. Just like you, she is learning to become a better parent. So don't make her feel bad when she doesn't look her best or has stains on her shirt or she forgot to get the diaper bag. If she forgets then you do it- you can step in and save the day.

Your Needs and Wants will come last

Yes, a child changes everything for you and your spouse. A baby is a life-changing event and if you ever thought things weren't going to change- you are in for a big surprise! Sexual relationships with your wife will change, boys-nights-out might happen once in a while, date nights will be rare, home cooked dinners will be different. Your routine will change and so will your spouse's. So be prepared for this rather than going through a cultural shock when the baby arrives. Of course, you'll only get the full effect of this when your child comes to the home, but it's always good to have some expectations ahead of time so you and your wife can prepare for the changes that will happen. Create timetables and put in tasks and events that you and her need to attend, doctor's appointments that you need to follow your wife for, feeding schedules and errand runs. Keep in mind for the better part of the first year when the baby comes, things will be different.

SHOW APPRECIATION

Your spouse or partner just pushed out a human the size of a watermelon from her body. She not only carried the baby for nine months but her physical appearance also changed. While fathers can still work out and keep a toned body, mother's bodies, on the other hand, go through a massive change to accommodate the life in her. Pregnancy is still one of the many marvels of life. If she's lucky to have a natural birth then great but some mothers also have to endure C-Sections. She has stretch marks, her belly is softer, and her skin might look a bit different. She will not only go through motherhood with the newborn, but she'll also have to go through the different changes in her body. SO show her appreciation whenever you can, as often as you can.

SPEND TIME TOGETHER

Sometime back when Chrissy Teigen and John Legend had a daughter, a week after the delivery, they went out on date night. Chrissy received a lot of backlash. John, on the other hand, didn't but what he did was to question why only his wife was shamed and not him, when in fact, both of them as parents went out for dinner. Women face much more adversities then men, unfortunately. So your wife might probably feel that a night out after a few weeks of delivering may not be appropriate, but this is where you come in. Spending quality time together is crucial no matter what the media or people around you say. If you feel your wife is in need of some r & r, then do something with her. It doesn't necessarily have to be a night out in town at some fancy restaurant- sometimes being apart so soon from your newborn might make her feel anxious. So take her out for brunch maybe at a nice café or even set a mani-pedi session at her favorite salon while you take care of the baby.

BE UNDERSTANDING

Ask her what is the best time she'd like to take a break for herself and then endeavor to give her that break as often as you can. She'll thank you immensely for this. Also, be understanding especially when she has any emotional bouts. She will feel ugly sometimes (the stretch marks can get to you) she will feel depressed sometimes and also yell at you for no apparent reason. Try to stay calm. Having a newborn is overwhelming and being a new mom is overwhelming, and you wouldn't necessarily understand what she's going through. But whatever you try to do, instead of fixing things just be there for her. All she needs is your understanding and not your solutions or judgment. Being understanding will also help calm situations at home especially when emotions tend to run a little bit different when the new baby comes, and there's a lot of crying one tiny little tyke.

BE PRESENT

Both as a father and husband. Your presence matters a lot to both mother and baby for many reasons such a shoulder to cry on, someone to talk to, someone to hug, and someone to laugh with. Don't pull away if she's distant- it's most likely she's tired or just focusing on the baby. Ask her if she's ok. Father's presence is very important to the newborn and the mother. Always remember that you are a team when it comes to bringing up your child together. Having both mother and father is always the best thing for the baby. No doubt there will be a lot of emotions going through between mother and father when the baby arrives but being responsible and being present and being understanding is what you need to be at this very moment in your life.

Of course, these are just some of the tips and advice that a new father can look into when you have a new addition to the family. There is plenty more advice than you can look for, but these are just some of the very basics that mothers want from the father. While it may be overwhelming, just remember that if you are determined to become a father and when that day happens, you will be looking forward to it and giving it all you got. Having a newborn will not only change your routine, but it will also make you become a better version of yourself.

CHAPTER 3: NEWBORN DEVELOPMENT

The first year of your newborn's life is the most exciting for any parent. You brought a human into this world, and now you get to watch your little one grow! In this chapter, we will look at the weeks of developments in a baby so you can watch your child's progress after reading this. Just remember that this is just a guideline- every baby develops differently at his or her own rate. Don't worry about whether your baby isn't doing what is described in this timeline. Every baby grows differently, and that is what makes them unique. But if you have any concerns about your child's development then discuss this with your pediatrician.

BABY'S FIRST YEAR

The human body is a beautiful thing. The newborn baby is another wonderful thing altogether. So the first 52 weeks one of the most exciting times for your baby and a very good time to learn new things. This is when bonds are established, and the baby adapts to the smell and sounds of her parents.

WEEK 1

In the first week, your newborn can already distinguish sounds and especially recognizes yours. The baby adjusts herself to the new world outside her mother's womb when she hears the familiar voices of her parents and those close to her.

This is a reassuring aspect for the baby so that she knows that she isn't alone in this world. This is why parental bonding at the first week is very important. The more you talk to her, kiss her, touch her, the more your baby will understand your words and your love and nurturing will come through.

WEEK 2

Your baby can now somewhat focus on objects that are about 8 to 14 inches away. This is just the distance of your baby's eyes and yours during feeding times. Baby's eyes are still not fully vivid yet, and they can only make our shadows. At this stage, they are more drawn to faces than they are with objects. So look at him while feeding him and this will also help him to practice focus. You can move your head slowly, sing songs and see if his eyes follow you. This also helps to track skills and builds his eye muscles.

WEEK 3

By the third week, you'll see a lot more body movement- it could still be random and jerky, but your baby will have a lot more control. She'll be able to snuggle as you hold her. She will reach out for your hand so reach out to her too because your scent will be calming and comforting. Allowing her fingers to curl around your index finger and doing small gentle movements is the most perfect and relaxing way for parents to bond with their child.

WEEK 4

Congratulations! Your baby is one-month-old! Your baby will be using more of her vocal cords in more ways than just crying. During this week, you'll hear a lot more cooing and gurgling and funny and cute sounds. This will happen more frequently when she sees mom or dad. Babies also learn sounds by mimicking, so this is a great way to start him on easy sounds like a cows' mooing or a cats' mewing. This is where babies will use more of their sounds, and you'd, of course, come running to see what it is.

WEEK 5

By the 5th week, your baby's movements will be a lot more fluid and smoother. His movements will also be more purposeful. Random, jerky moves transition into smooth and purposeful moves. At this point, you can do simple exercises with your baby like moving his hands or putting him up into a sitting position. Remember that you want gentle and light moving because baby's limbs are still fragile. Remember to always support the head. You would be able to do plenty of different small movements with your baby by the 5th week. You can even play with your baby in front of a mirror and mimic whatever he is doing. As the baby gets older this will be a fun way of learning new things and different movements. Always remember to touch and speak to him to maximize on your bonding sessions with your baby.

WEEK 6 – WEEK 8

Week 6 will open up another new array of changes for your baby. At this point, your baby will also be showing gummy grins which will be his first genuine smile! You'll see his eyes brightening and his mouth moving upwards to a smile each time something attracts his attention or he sports a familiar face. By smiling back and cooing at him, you'll encourage his reactions and probably see more smiles. At this stage, you are indirectly teaching him that his actions will cause reactions.

Your baby's senses will also improve, and she will also start making sense of her senses. Her tastes in color will develop too, where she will look at bright colors and 3D objects. This is a great time to have a mobile hanging above her crib so that she can follow it and smile. Neck muscles also get stronger, and your baby would be able to lift his head at about 45 degrees.

WEEK 9 –WEEK 11

By this time, your baby's tiny little world would be alive with music. Literally, any sound will fascinate her especially high tones. She will also look intently at you when you speak so this is a good time to read to her. It will build her vocabulary with words. She will also be able to recognize her parent's face from a small group of people. Any indication such as the widening of eyes or a gurgle is an indication that she is familiar with the person in front of her. Your baby's sleeping patterns also change here. She is more anxious to learn about the world around her and the family she is with. She will sleep less and be awake more. This is where you must establish sleeping routines.

WEEK 12- 14

Your baby's hands will be his most favorite thing to focus on at this point. He would be able to bring his hands together, even sort of clap (especially if he's seen you doing this before) he will put them in his mouth, and he will start exploring more with his hands. At this point, you can start introducing to him rubber toys. Make sure they are non-toxics and safe for babies at 12 to 14 weeks. With more established sleeping patterns, you will have more time to sleep as well. Keep talking to your baby, repeating words and syllables especially ones that are connected to eating and sleeping. Rattles and dangling toys will be her best friends for now, and they will also help her hand-eye coordination.

4 MONTHS OLD

Your baby is reaching four months old! Your baby by this time will be more mobile. She'll start rolling over and eventually learn to master these rolls to the direction that she chooses. Make sure her bed is never on a high surface and the crib is well protected. By this time, she is also a lot stronger and does a lot of crawling. Make sure you are always in her range of vision when you talk to her, even getting down to floor level to be with her. Your baby is by this time, already entertaining everyone around her with her bouts of gurgling and cooing, movement of hands and also laughter. Her eyesight will also be sharp by now, and she'll use more of her eyes and hands to learn and play with herself. Keep her toys educational so that it can improve cognitive reception as well as hand-eye coordination. You will also hear her say words by this time. Usually 'daa daa'. At 4 months old, point to her eyes or mouth or nose and pronounce the name. While she may not be able to say it, she will remember this and this will become part of her first vocabulary.

6 MONTHS

Your baby has reached half a milestone in his life! At this point, he's a charmer but is more selective and wary of whom he smiles to. No stranger gets a smile unless he is familiar with the person. At this point, your baby may not be very comfortable when in groups of adults so you get to decide who gets to hold him and who doesn't. But more often, your baby will decide that for himself by crying. When this happens, then take him away and establish a goodbye to give your baby a sense of security. From here onwards, there will be several things that you need to create because your baby will be able to remember certain things, respond to certain things. Sleeping and eating routines must be more evident now because it will only make things easier as your baby grows older.

Be careful of choking hazards because your baby would be curious to pick anything that he sees and put it into his mouth. At this point, you can introduce more different games such as peek-a-boos and finding objects that you've hidden in your hand. Blocks are also a great play tool to have at this time.

10 MONTHS OLD

Can you believe it! Your tiny little tyke is ten months old! Your baby by now is already imitating your actions such as combing his hair. He will also start learning how to walk, taking small steps. This is a perfect time to take him out to the park and teach him to walk. Be careful though because your baby is still not ready to walk without your help. Establish a bedtime story with your baby and read something things for him to hear. Let him touch the book, look at the pages and point to him when you say words. Your baby will be wobbling so fast you might as well cancel your fitness club membership because you'll get the workout you need. Continue bonding with your child here. Take him to parks and to family gatherings. Introduce him to the pool and make sure he has all the safety around him.

If your child has not shown any signs of walking, don't worry- some kids take up to 16 to 19 months to walk.

Your baby is also ready for the baby chair, and she can already start slightly feeding herself so let her do this if she wants to. Of course, despite want to feed her own self, she will dribble and mess her place up. Let her. This will develop her self-esteem and also help her to master her motor skills.

1 YEAR OLD

Look how far we've come! Happy birthday to your not-so-little bundle of joy! By this time, she will have developed more words on her own, and her first words could be mama or dada! Continue teaching, talking, bonding and establishing rules and boundaries, routines and schedules so your growing baby will know the rules of the house and connecting with her parents and siblings.

This timeline only serves as a guideline on the early developments of a baby till he or she reaches one year old. Again, not every baby is the same and not every baby will go through the same growth as explained in this timeline.

If you are worried about your child's development, the best thing to do is to take your child to a pediatrician and get their feedback and advice. Sometimes, parents worry too much about their child's development especially when people around them make comments or nosy aunts and uncles point out why isn't the child doing so and so, or the child is supposed to act a certain way. Rest assured that different children develop differently. No matter what, always consult a doctor or pediatrician and continue giving your baby the support, encouragement and nurturing that he or she requires.

CHAPTER 4: NEWBORN & INFANT NUTRITION

There is plenty of advice out there for new parents when it comes to infant nutrition and any parent can certainly get confused or worried that they might not be giving their child the best possible. However, infant nutrition isn't entirely complex. In this chapter, we will look at some advice from Precision Nutrition and look at a simple guideline to ensure that your infant is off to a healthy and wonderful start.

Infancy, the first year of line is a primary time for necessary growth and changes that take place in the body. What we eat when we are babies influences our long term body weight, health, immune system as well as metabolic state and aging.

Here is a simple guideline of what your child needs to be eating, at least for the first year of their lives:

THE FIRST 6 MONTHS

Breast milk is the best for newborns. For the first six months of their lives, babies can be fed exclusively breast milk because it contains the optimal nutrient mixture for infants. Breast milk has everything the growing baby needs such as antibodies, antimicrobial elements, enzymes as well as anti-inflammatory characteristics together with essential fatty acids which are essential for brain development.

86

Breast feeding keeps your newborn developing and growing well and it also helps their immune system get stronger so that any diseases, such as gastrointestinal and respiratory infections are kept at bay. Breastfeeding keeps the immune system tough and it only gets better as the baby grows older.

There are many benefits for breastfeeding. One of it is that is stimulates the release of beneficial hormones for the baby such as oxytocin and prolactin. More interesting is the fact that breast feeding helps the mother to lose weight gained during pregnancy but more importantly, breast feeding is encouraged very much by organizations like "WHO", who say that breastfeeding helps the bonding process.

Not every mother takes to breast feeding like its' the most natural thing to do. Some find it hard and some find breastfeeding painful. In the case of painful or difficult breastfeeding, consult a midwife or better yet, your own mother. Mothers can also get some advice from lactation consultants who will teach them proper techniques to help a mother breastfeed successfully.

While breastfeeding is the best thing for the baby, never feel guilty if you cannot breastfeed exclusively. Many mother experience varying degrees of difficulty when it comes to breastfeeding.

Some mothers on the other hand are unable to breastfeed due to health problems or if they are under certain medication. Whatever it is, don't worry about it- just do your best. And don't worry even more that your baby isn't getting the right nutrition if they are exclusively formula-fed. Formula-fed babies do just fine.

Whatever approach you are going for, always remember to speak to your pediatrician about it especially when choosing the right formula for your baby. Essentially, here are a few guidelines to remember whether breastfeeding or formula-feeding:

- Avoid soy-based formulas
- Remember what you eat will be passed into the breast milk. Your baby eats what you eat.
- Limit alcohol and caffeine as well as any toxin exposure
- Eat organic as much as possible and make sure to clean your fruits and veggies
- Avoid eating seafood because it mercury is linked to brain damage

Moms must remember to eat nutritiously while she is pregnant and when she is breastfeeding. Breast milk provides all the essential nutrients an infant needs for the first six vital months of its life. Here is a quick guideline on what babies need to develop their muscles, bones and brain development. Some of these nutrients can be via supplementation:

VITAMIN D

Vitamin D is naturally received from the sun. In some parts of the world, Vitamin D is low because of the weather and that leaves some mothers deficient in Vitamin D during pregnancy and breastfeeding. Research has also shown that preemies are also found to have low levels of vitamin D. To increase this, the American Academy of Pediatrics (AAP) suggests a daily vitamin D intake of 400IU for all breast-fed infants, starting immediately after birth. Formula fed infants once they have reached at least 30 ounces of formula per day, supplementation of Vitamin D can be discontinues. Breast fed infants are encourage to be given vitamin D supplements will they are one year old.

For mothers that already have sufficient vitamin D levels in her, this can be passed on to the baby. Again, anything that you are considering firstly checking with your doctor or pharmacist or pediatrician. Test your vitamin D levels and then speak to your doctor to ensure the best and safest option for your newborn.

VITAMIN B12

A mother who is exclusively vegan and only eats plant-based must supplement vitamin B12 for her infant. Again, checking your levels of B12 is essential because if you are deficit then your baby is deficit as well.

IRON

The fetus will receive iron from the mother's blood while it is in the womb. However, breast milk doesn't have much iron but it is well absorbed by the infant. Iron can last in the infant's body up till 6 months of age therefore the infant will not require further iron supplementation unless he or she is a premature. Formula fed infants will also be able to get the require iron.

PROBIOTICS

The first form of bacteria introduced to the infant is through the birth canal because while the baby is in the womb, it is a sterile environment. The bacterium from the birth canal colonizes the mucous membranes as well as the gastrointestinal tract. Don't worry though- this is perfectly normal and just as how Nature intended it to be. In a C-section, this bacterial colonization doesn't happen as smoothly as possible. When this doesn't happen, the baby will often face issues later on related to respiratory, gastrointestinal as well as ear-nose-throat infections. It may also lower the baby's immune system.

Not to fret though, with the advances of modern medicine, parents can prevent this by supplementing the infant with probiotic formula. Your pediatrician will know what to subscribe.

Usually, breast milk or formula already has the required amount of fluids necessary for the baby to keep them hydrated. However, infants can still be dehydrated especially in extreme conditions such as when the baby has fever or is vomiting or when the temperature is hot. Diarrhea can also cause rehydration and this can be solved by adding a little sugar and salt to the water to make a simple electrolyte solution.

Your baby's urine is a good indication of how hydrated she is. Over-hydration results in clear urine. You want something in between. Take your body cues as a measure of how dark or light your baby's urine is.

THE NEXT 6 TO 12 MONTHS

At this point you can start introducing semi-solid food to your baby's diet. Most infants still can't digest foods and they can only do this when they have grown to a weight that is double their birth weight. Usually when your baby is ready which is about the six month mark, they are also physically ready to hold their heads up, sit in a high chair or open their mouths when food is given. They will also be able to swallow.

In addition to breast milk, offer them solid foods. Don't make this a replacement; rather it is more of a supplement. These solid foods are still in a liquid more but a little bit more consistent than milk. Take your time in introducing solids because there is no need to rush. In addition to breast milk, feed your baby semi-solid food every once in 4 days. You can see how your baby responds and reacts to these various introductions.

If your baby's body responds negatively such as having respiratory problems, skin rashes or GI issues, stop the solids and wait another 1 to 3 months before reintroducing them. Speak to your pediatrician about these signs.

SOLID FOOD TIMELINE

STEP 1- INTRODUCING RICE CEREALS

Rice cereals with breast milk or formula is among the most common first foods most parents will introduce to their children no matter where in the world you are. This is a well-tolerated food item with little or no allergy at all.

STEP 2- VEGGIES

When introducing vegetables to your infant, puree them to its easier to swallow. Sweet potatoes, squashes, carrots and beets are great to cook and pulverize.

STEP 3- FRUITS

Fruits are much sweeter than vegetables so do not make this your first solid food introduction. Also, babies will have a lower tolerance to digest fructose properly so keep your fruit feeding to a moderate level and avoid high-fiber fruits such as prunes, peach, pears, and papayas.

STEP 4- HIGH PROTEIN FOODS

Finely chopped meats, lentils, green peas and mashed beans are a great introduction when your baby hits 7 to 8 months old.

12 MONTHS AND OLDER

By the time your toddler turns one year old, he would have pretty much achieved a more robust palette. One year olds can eat solid food, but still somewhat soft in a way. You can start your child on a diet that consists of these items:

- avocado
- tree nuts
- string beans
- asparagus
- puréed fresh fruit
- egg yolk
- mashed lentils/beans
- meat, chicken, or mild-tasting fish

All of the above can be finely chopped or mashed or pureed. Meat can be shredded into tiny bits so that it is easier on the infant's gums and will prevent any choking.

Be cautious of fish though. While it can be eaten by 1 year old infants, experts warn against consuming too much of shellfish at such an early stage because it can cause allergic reactions. A good thing to do is to wait till the child is older. Other things to hold on first would be egg whites or even whole eggs, peanuts, dairy milk, soy and wheat.

When introducing new food items into your child's diet, just look out for any reactions before adding on anything else. Most kids to just well with many of these foods, but a careful watch is always good when it comes to food intake.

TIPS ON GETTING YOUR INFANT TO EAT

Feeding time can be a challenge as your child grows up. As their palate becomes more and more sophisticated, their likes and dislikes will also become more evident. So what do you do? Here are some tips to help you out with feeding time:

1. ADD VARIETY WHILE PREGNANT

What you eat during pregnancy will set the tone of what your baby will tolerate and like. The native cuisine of your country will without a doubt be something your baby will be drawn to when older because that is what the mother has been eating. Your baby will continue the healthy eating habits that you had while pregnant, so long as you do not introduce fast food and additives too early in childhood.

2. CREATE AN EATING SCHEDULE

Establishing eating patterns and schedules will help your infant adjust to breakfast, lunch and dinner. Also, take note of when your child is most hungry as this will help the parent introduce new foods easily like broccoli, carrots, pumpkin and so on.

3. ADD SOME SWEETNESS TO THE DISH

We humans are born with the natural inclination for sweet things because it is nature's way of adding in energy rich foods into our diet. Naturally sweet foods such as sweet potato and fruits can be added together with less-sweet food items.

4. AVOID PROCESSED SUGAR

Whatever your baby eats now will affect their preferences as an adult. As much as possible, avoid processed sugar and this is especially evident in commercial baby foods together with commercial fruit purees and juices. Avoid honey as well because it contains bacteria that the baby's immune system cannot handle yet.

5. KEEP A FOOD ROUTINE

Infants sometimes refuse to eat a certain food and that's all fine because they aren't used to it. Leave it out for a bit and then bring the food back into the feeding routine. Over time you'll realize that they are more relaxed at eating it.

Sometimes, it is always good to let the baby explore food options. Eat with them and sometimes they will show signs of interest of the food that's on your plate. This is totally find- just make sure what they are reaching for is something they can it. If not, make it fine so they can chew it.

6. ALWAYS EAT WHOLE FOODS

Do not force-feed your child. Infants will know how much they need so if they stop eating, do not keep forcing them, unless you see some different changes in their eating patterns. Also, do not introduce any kind of processed food before whole foods as this will compromise the infant's gut flora. Always look at your baby's hunger levels and their food preferences while you continue to expand their palate with more high-quality and nutritious foods. The hunger cues from your infant are important to parents- infants will want to eat when they are hungry and stop when they are full.

While it is good to establish eating routines, remember that you can also bend the rules a little bit because there is no point in pressuring your baby into a set schedule especially in their early days or wake them up for feeding at night. Babies will have a rhythm which you will know, so stick to that for a bit.

7. COMMUNICATE WITH YOUR BABY

Learning hunger cues from them is part of their rhythm. Watch your baby 'sign' for when she's hungry or when she's full or if she wants something. Babies can tell so just make sure you watch- this is also part of bonding.

8. WEIGHT GAIN

Here is a rough guide of how much your baby should gain weight. Remember, every baby is different so always consult your pediatrician on this.

- First 3 months- your baby can gain about 2 pounds/month
- At 6 months- your baby gains at least 1 pound/month
- At 9 months- your baby gains less than 1 pound/month

Babies are usually weighed every time they go to the doctor and this is often enough on most normal circumstances.

MAKING YOUR OWN INFANT MEALS

The most healthy baby food out there is the one made at home. Making baby food is super simple because all you need is fresh ingredients and food and a food processor or blender. Once you start mashing and chopping and pureeing, you help your baby expand his palate. Make baby food simple so you know exactly what he's eating. Infant food must be blended or mashed well to avoid any foods that can cause choking. As always, follow basic food rules like washing your hands, refrigerating or heating food properly and immediate discard any food that is compromised or has expired.

97

INFANT NUTRIENT REQUIREMENTS

Here is a general guideline for nutrient intake for infants from 6 months to 2 years of age.

FATS

Infants and children need plenty of the good fat which is saturated, monounsaturated and omega-3 fats. Where do you find them? Here is a list of food items that contain healthy fat:

- avocado;
- coconut;
- butter
- high-fat dairy;
- meat;
- egg
- fatty fish from healthy animals
- Nuts, seeds and nut butters (make your own nut butter- these products can come later)

Essential fats are crucial in overall health but mostly they help in the development of the eyes, brain and nervous system.

IRON

Iron is important for neurological, cognitive and behavioral development. Iron is usually introduced around 6 months of age. Here are some iron-rich foods:

- leafy greens
- orange-fleshed squash
- figs
- raisins
- nuts & seeds
- lentils
- artichokes
- peas & lima beans
- potatoes
- chicken or beef liver (try sneaking a little bit in to blended meat)
- red meat
- chicken and duck
- fish

Do not go overboard with iron. Also, do not give babies any soy, almond, help, or cow's milk especially when they are still breastfeeding.

ZINC

Zinc is essential for cell development. Foods that are rich in zinc include:

- peas & beans
- nuts & seeds
- napa cabbage

- hearts of palm
- sun-dried tomatoes
- cocoa powder
- meat, poultry (especially darker cuts), fish
- cheese

HYDRATION

Apart from the above, make sure your baby is well hydrated. After six months, you can slowly start introducing fruit juices made from fresh fruits and vegetables. Avoid commercial grade ones because they contain sugar and sugar will lead to your infant developing cravings for sweet things which will lead to cavities and body fat. Avoid any artificial sweeteners too. Stick with water most of the time and give home-made fruit juices only on special occasions.

Recommendations:

For the next 17 years of your child's life- you are in charge of it which (well, maybe lesser as he gets older). But for the first few years, you can control what your child eats so give your infant the best start.

If you can, continue breastfeeding even after the age of 1. Most experts recommend breastfeeding till the child is 2 years old. Supplements should be checked with your doctor before administering and this is usually for vitamin D and B12 after they reach 2 months of age.

After 6 months, start introducing your infant to solid foods such as rice cereal, pureed vegetables and then followed by fruits and protein-dense foods. Introduce one new food at a time and see how your infant reacts to it.

Always opt for whole foods and do not give them processed or commercial grade foods. Cook as often as you can and prepare home-cooked meals. This will develop a taste preference which will carry on till adulthood.

Be aware of your baby's hunger signals and food preferences. Patiently add variety into her diet and adjust mealtime schedules so that it accommodates her hunger levels. Go as organic as much as you can and minimize and added sugars which includes fruit juices and processed foods.

For the first size months of your baby's life, breast milk provides the adequate amount of fluid but after this, add water to their diet. Avoid any soy or cow or processed milks.

While parenting is hard, just try your best to give your child the best you can. Nobody is perfect so do not try to be a perfect mother or perfect father.

Chapter 5: Early Education for the Toddler

Every parent wants the best for their children especially when it comes to what they eat and their education. You must be wondering when is a good time to start your child on the ABCs and 123s. The truth is, educating your infant starts the minute he is born. Everything you do, everything you say and the time spent with him is all new things for him, and he will learn this as he grows older.

For example, a father who takes his daughter to the park is already teaching her valuable lessons. For one, there's trust. Two, the father talks to the child, points out all the colors and shapes that she sees- this is all part of educating the child. Sure it may not be in a classroom setting but there are many ways of educating a child and in the confines of a classroom isn't the only way. When you talk, your child absorbs all this information, expanding his vocabulary and at the same time identifying the things around him. Education also happens when the family eats together, prays together or reads together and even spends time together. Teaching also happens during bedtime- when you teach your child to wash himself, brush his teeth and when you read him a bedtime story.

All these things are stuff that cannot be taught in school because, at the end of the day, the world we live in is a source of education for toddler and heck, even adults. Erin Seaton, lecturer at the Department of Education at Tufts University in Massachusetts, says that "Toddlers love to master new concepts, so it's the perfect time to lay the foundation for future skills like reading and counting,"

The key to toddler education is playing off from your child's interests. Have plenty of fun doing everyday activities is what will make him interested. Add in colors and sounds and role-playing and you have a kid that is vibrant, energetic and eager to learn.

Here are some of the first few things that you can teach your toddler once she has reached the age of one:

LEARNING LETTERS

Some of the simplest ways to learn the letters of the alphabet are by teaching her to spell her name. By doing this, your child will be able to recognize the letters that make up her name and to reinforce this, have her name displayed throughout your home such as on her bedroom door, on her baby high chair and even on the fridge. By saying out loud each letter, your child will know how to say it and how it sounds. Remember how we were taught the alphabet in school - say and repeat it? Do it exactly like this.

ENCOURAGE READING

Whenever you are anywhere with your child, point out words and letters on signage, boxes and places you frequently visit with her. Sherril English, the education professor at Southern Methodist University, says that saying things out loud will help our child think of words that rhyme, which will then improve her vocabulary. Remember to speak slowly, enunciate clearly as you read your words.

KNOWING NUMBERS

Just like reading, counting also requires you to count it out for your toddler so that she may be able to recite them as they grow older. Listening to you say the numbers will make it easier for her to catch the pronunciation and say it on her own eventually. While toddlers can somehow say the words when they turn one or two years old, they will probably not be able to count until they reach preschool. But by repeating and saying numbers out loud, they are able to recognize these numbers. Try buttoning up your toddler's dress or shirt and say 'one, two, three buttons'. Things like that will help them identify numbers. Use your fingers when counting too so that your toddler will be able to copy you.

SHOW & TELL

Teaching your child early mathematics even before she goes off to preschool involves observation and comparison. Parents must know that toddlers are master copiers and sorters-babies and toddlers learn fast by observing and copying so take advantage of that. What you can do is get your child to group her toys accordingly- blocks in the basket, stuffed animals in a box and same colored toys in one drawer. Your toddler will learn how to coordinate things and best of all- you didn't have to clean up after her. Your child will learn a lot by observing you so instill good manners in her as well like saying 'please' and 'thank you'.

HAVE FUN LEARNING!

Toddlers love colors and shapes. Get a shape book to that you can help your child color inside the shapes and tell her what these shapes are. Again, spell it out so she identifies the letters as well. You can also draw basic shapes on a piece of paper or while flipping through magazines or newspapers, cut out different shapes and tell your child what these shapes are. If you are out for a walk with her, point out at street signs and ask her what it is- you'd be surprised she'll be able to identify them. Point at a round tire or a square window or even a rectangular brick- ask her what they are. All these different activities increases bonding between parent and child.

You can also use cookie cutters to help your toddler identify shapes. Even food can be used to help your child identify shapes such as squares of a sandwich or cookies that are rectangular or round, look at pancakes, slices of cheese and even bread. You can even create a shape chart for her and label each shape so she'll learn from memory as well. These are excellent tips to get your child to learn and identify shapes.

COLORS

Colors are another fun thing to learn. This can be done with food or even art projects. Get your toddler to do finger painting with you or go on a scavenger hunt to find for different color things such as a red brick or a green garden hose, a yellow flower, the blue of the sky and even a green leaf. You'd get your child to learn about the outdoors and colors at the same time. When getting your child to clean up after himself, use descriptive language such as 'Can you please put in the blue ball into the yellow box?'. During mealtimes, you can ask him if he'd like a red apple or a yellow banana or if he would like green grapes. Identifying the colors with the food also helps the child quickly equate different items in the household with its colors. All these different things sets the foundation for your child. Learning doesn't need to start when the child starts pre-school. It can start right at home. In fact, research shows that children with a strong set of attitudes and skills gives them a head start in school and helps them learn faster. They will be much better equipped to take advantage of the educational opportunities present in the schooling environment. Some learning skills come naturally to kids while some can be developed through supportive schooling environment.

TIPS TO BUILD LEARNING SKILLS

1. Let kids choose

Allow your children to make simple choices such as what they would like to wear or what they would like to have for a snack. This also builds confidence in children.

2. Help them finish what they started

Not only is this a good training grown for them mentally, allowing children to finish what they started allows them to indulge in the experience of satisfaction. Give them support when they need it but never take over completely.

3. Encourage creativity

Kids explore things and ask a lot of questions so try using different materials or expose them to different kinds of experience.

4. Don't rush

While we all want our children to get a head-start in life, we as parents must also remember not to rush things. Some children need extended periods of time to understand the activities and experience it at their own pace. This is a very important foundation of learning.

ALWAYS GIVE POSITIVE ENCOURAGEMENT

Children have varying levels of absorbing information, and all children are eager to learn, but parents cannot be too critical if they do not achieve in doing things. By being critical, we may suppress their eagerness to learn particularly in the elementary stage. Comment and encouragement them but do not overdo the praise (it might result in over-confidence). Your toddler is still in the stages of discovering the world so while he's at it, don't discourage him.

They will explore and use their senses to learn everything they can. Keep a watchful eye, help them when necessary and commend them whenever the situation calls for it. If they get it wrong or misbehave, that's when you come in and teach them how to do something or teach them how it's done right. As much as possible, use non-verbal communication and physical strategies to teach your toddlers because again, they follow by example. Your simple gestures and sounds and speeches can help them understand what you are trying to say clearly.

METHODS OF TEACHING CHILDREN

METHOD ONE - THROUGH INITIATIVE, ENGAGEMENT AND PERSISTENCE

- Using simple language and indicating preferences through non-verbal communication such as pointing to an apple and pushing a bunch of grapes away
- Focusing a child's attention to interesting sights and sounds such as reading a farm animal book to a child and making sounds of the animals
- Show pleasure when a child completes a task such as putting away his toys of coloring inside the lines
- Your child may want to help with adult tasks such as turning the page of the book or helping to peel the bananas.

METHOD TWO – PIQUING CURIOSITY AND EAGERNESS TO LEARN

- Get children to participate actively in sensory experience such as tasting, touching, playing
- Kids also point to objects that interest them so parents can answer by saying a single word. Children will eventually learn to combine these words when asking simple questions
- Kids also show physical and vocal pleasure when they discover something that intrigues them such as when they pick up bells and it rings.
- For parents, if you know something will interest them, and then try to get your child more exposed to these items. For example, some kids create an interest in dinosaurs or the

stars so take them to museums or the planetarium to expand their interest- just get ready for more questions!

PROBLEM-SOLVING & REASONING

- As your child grows older, they will employ various physical strategies to reach simple tasks and goals such as putting boxes back into their shelves or even pushing a cart through a door
- Kids will also use gestures with simple language when they are two years old to get help such as when they are stuck or if they want to get into a high chair.
- Your kid will also thoughtfully work towards creating gestures that will improve his language skills and exploration. This would be a great time to teach him other ways of problem solving. For example, teach your how to peel a banana the right way or how to turn a book without crumpling the pages. These simple gestures teach them better problem-solving skills.

INVENTION AND IMAGINATION

- Every child has a vivid imagination! Their imagination is so great that it helps with their creativity. They are able to play with mundane objects but yet feel so fascinated by it. They can pick up a building block and use it as a phone, take a ball and use it as a car- the thing is toddlers use the most simplest of objects to entertain themselves.

- Their use of objects is vivid based on their expanse their imagination such as using a saucepan over their heads like a helmet.

CHAPTER 6: DISCIPLINING TODDLERS

The saying goes 'Spare the Rod and spoil the child'- it's easier said than done. Baby boomers can tell you that the rod was the go-to disciplining technique back in the 60s. Many parents of today's generation would rather not take the rod out and that is totally understandable.

Techniques have changed throughout the years on the best ways of disciplining children and yes it isn't easy to discipline your kid. But in this chapter, we will look at keeping the peace and changing both the behavior of the parent as well as child for the better.

FIXING BAD BEHAVIOR

Nothing drives a parent crazy than hearing their children whining and complaining and of course pointing fingers at the other sibling. From the whining and complaining then comes the 'smack-down' between siblings. As much as our children throw temper tantrums, we also have to look at the way parents handle these arguments.

Bernard Percy, a child consultant in Los Angeles says that focusing on what the child has done wrong will only increase arguments and bad behavior conduct. Children's annoying tendencies tend to bring out the worst in parents and then parents start yelling. So it makes you wonder- how can your children change their negative habits if you can't change yours? Here are some tips to work on fixing bad behavior in children:

TIP 1: DON'T REACT

Again, easier said than done. Sometimes you just need to bite your tongue. Ed Christophersen, a clinical child psychologist at Children's Mercy Hospitals and Clinics, in Kansas City, Missouri says giving your children new policies will help calm them down during tantrums and mood swings. Parents are advised to not respond to misbehavior. So when your child gets into a moment of hysterics and tantrums, tell that that you are not going to listen or see them unless they stop their bickering.

Your child would obviously continue their tantrums, screaming at the top of their lungs just so they can get your attention but don't back down. Don't hand them a candy so that they'd keep quiet. Let your child continue because eventually they'll realize that whining and crying will lose its appeal. Eventually.

TIP 2: STAY POSITIVE

The tantrums will continue because behaviors don't change overnight. Author of 'Thinking Your Way to Happy! Robin H.C says that when you label a child as naughty or aggressive or childish, you are putting them into a self-fulfilling prophecy.

So next time, say positive things. Tell your child something positive so that they can live up to it.

If your child throws a tantrum of not finding the right soldiers for her fortress, tell her that she's good at making things so find something else. Encourage the younger or older sibling to help out. When this happens, give credit where it's due. Commend your child for the good things they do.

TIP 3: WALK THE TALK

If you want to change your child's behavior, you should change yours. You as a parent should be the model of good behavior because you need to lead by example. So if you do not want your children whining, stop whining yourself. In fact, stop nagging incessantly and this advice goes for both parents-fathers and mothers. If your kids dawdle to get ready for school, give them a time limit so they know how long they have to get themselves out the door. Also, remember positive labeling.

If your kids whine too much at the table, give them the 5 minute rule- eat for 5 minutes, talk for 5 minutes otherwise no TV or dessert.

Establishing certain rules helps you maintain the calm. It helps you remain calm too in order to give you some time to assess how you would want to react to any tantrums and issues that may rise. Remember that your goal is to remain calm in the face of adversity. Do not do the things you do not want your kids to act or say or behave. Always try a positive approach to any issues that may rise and above all, both father and mother act as a team.

TIP 4: CONFIRM BEFORE DISCIPLINING

Oftentimes when our children do something wrong, break something, pound each other or go on a tantrum, we are quick to wrong the party that did the mistake without validating or enquiring or investigating.

Gary M. Unrah the author of 'Unleashing the Power of Parental Love' says that kids throw tantrums or act out for a reason- as everyone does. Gary says that telling your kids the feelings of why they have misbehaved will give them fair play. This will make your child feel understood and accepted, and eventually bring them towards being disciplined.

For example, if your child tore her favorite book, instead of saying "Next time make sure where you keep your books, you know better than that to leave them lying around carelessly" instead say 'It is a pity you tore your book, you must be sad; a good thing to do is to keep them back at the bookshelves when you are done reading'.

If your child is angry, tell them that yes, they have the right to be angry. But send them to their room for a time-out because they need to learn the consequences of their actions and also learn to manage their anger. You'd be surprised after the time out, they will come out much calmer and have no sulking. Remember, feelings first and discipline second is probably the best trick a parent can have in their arsenal of disciplining their children. Have the patience to implement this rule as it will take you a long way.

TIP 5: MAKE YOUR EXPECTATIONS CLEAR

For all parents all around the world no matter what your cultural background is, your reaction to your kids heavily depends on your mood for the day or time. Bertie Bregman, the chief of family medicine at the New York Presbyterian Hospital advices parents to be consistent and make their expectations from their children clear to avoid outbursts. For example, one of your methods of educating your child on their tantrums is repeating your mantra to them. If your child whines about not having their chosen Happy Meal toy, then tell them 'you get what you get and 5 year olds don't whine'. Keep repeating this mantra till they have this set in their heads. To be satisfied with what you have at the moment and don't simply whine just because you didn't get something you wanted to first time.

TIP 6: CHANGE THE RULES OF THE GAME

Sometimes, boundaries have to readjusted, according to Catherine Hickem, author of Regret Free Parent. She suggests changing the rules from time to time. For example if you find yourself having to deal with your children's tantrums each time you make dinner, you might want to try taking away the remote on one day. Yes there will be havoc but you just need to deal with it, close one eye and one ear and get on with your job. Keep doing this for some time till your children get the hang of it. But if they tantrums start again, change your tactic. Try instead not allowing them to watch TV at all and instead work on their own projects like coloring or block building. You'd fine that over time, your children will learn to not throw any tantrums when you are making dinner and they would learn to occupy themselves when the TV is turned off or when you've taken away the remote.

Changing the rules of the game when it comes to your children will teach to them that they cannot simply whine or sulk when things do not go their way. It will also teach them to respect someone else's time and more importantly, make them independent to think of other ways of entertaining themselves apart from just watching TV. In other words, you also reduce their TV time.

TIP 7: CHILLING OUT

While a mother or father's job is never done (or more importantly a mother's job does not end), it is also good to teach them that everyone needs some rest and that includes mommy and daddy. Every Saturday or Sunday, take time off as a family and leave the house to go to somewhere where the kids can have fun and the parents can relax and by this, it doesn't have to be a holiday destination. Do things as a family and go to the park, spend the time playing catch, reading books, having races and basically enjoying each other's companies. Even better, make it a family ritual of having a picnic every Sunday. Pack some sandwiches, take the ball, have a good time away from the house, away from home responsibilities and leave the stress at home.

A short trip to a park or the gardens or even lunch at a restaurant helps the family connect again, talk to each other and enjoy each other's company.

This are just some of the ways to help in disciplining children and remember, when disciplining them, we as parents much change our ways too. Less shouting more listening, less outburst more reasoning. Family time every once a week, having at least one meal a day together as a family as well as doing parent-child things together also help in disciplining the child.

CONCLUSION

Essentially, parenting is the journey of encouraging and supporting the emotional, social, financial, intellectual and also the physical development of a child from infancy all right through to adulthood. Wikipedia describes parenting as the process of raising a child that is not related to the biological relationship. So meaning even If you aren't biologically related to the child, you can still parent them.

Apart from the biological or non-biological parents, the child also has other influences in parenting usually the older sibling, grandparents, an aunt or uncle or a legal guardian.

Hopefully, this book has shed some light for parents and would-be parents on the various aspects of parenting in the simplest way possible.

42957700R00069

Made in the USA
San Bernardino, CA
12 December 2016